TABLE OF CONTENTS

Loss, in its myriad forms, casts a long shadow over the human experience, touching every life with its nuanced and sometimes unexpected presence. To truly understand grief, we must embark on a journey to explore the diverse landscapes of loss, recognizing that its manifestations are as varied as the kaleidoscope of human connections and aspirations. — 8

DISCLAIMER

The information provided in this book, "Tears That Heal:Honouring grief,embracing hope in the face of loss" is for general informational purposes only. The content is not intended to be a substitute for professional advice.

The author and publisher of this book make no representations or warranties of any kind, express or implied, about the completeness, accuracy, reliability, suitability, or availability of the information contained herein. Any reliance you place on such information is strictly at your own risk.

COPYRIGHT

Copyright © [2024] by [Mercy Grace]

TEARS THAT HEALS

HONOURING GRIEF, EMBRACING HOPE IN THE FACE OF LOSS

Mercy Grace

INTRODUCTION: THE JOURNEY WITHIN

In the profound tapestry of human existence, few threads weave a more intricate and challenging pattern than the emotions stirred by loss. "Tears That Heal: Honouring Grief, Embracing Hope in the Face of Loss" is an exploration into the depths of these emotions, a guidebook for those traversing the delicate path of grief, and a beacon of hope for the weary hearts in search of healing.

This introduction serves as the gateway to "The Journey Within," inviting readers to embark on a personal odyssey into the realms of sorrow and resilience. Here, we acknowledge the universal nature of grief, recognizing that it is an emotion that touches each of us in unique and profound ways. Through an empathetic lens, we delve into the multifaceted nature of grief, understanding it not as a mere reaction to loss, but as a transformative journey that can lead to profound personal growth.

Within these pages, we will unravel the layers of grief, exploring its varied landscapes and shedding light on the different types of loss that shape our lives. As we embark on this exploration, we invite readers to reflect on their own experiences, recognizing that the path of grief is as individual as the person who walks it.

"The Journey Within" is not a solitary expedition; it is a collective voyage shared by those who have weathered the storm of loss and emerged with newfound strength. We will honour the memories of loved ones, acknowledging that they live on in the stories we tell and the rituals we create. Through the art of expressing grief, whether through words, art, or music, we discover the healing power of self-expression.

This introduction sets the stage for the chapters that follow, each offering a nuanced perspective on grief and loss. It is an invitation to explore coping strategies, navigate the impact of grief on relationships, and ultimately find hope amidst the darkness. As we embark on this journey together, let us recognize that tears, far from being a sign of weakness, can be powerful catalysts for healing, shaping a path toward renewed purpose and a life that honors the profound impact of those we have lost.

UNDERSTANDING GRIEF

DEFINING GRIEF: A MULTIFACETED EMOTION

Grief, an emotion that reverberates through the chambers of the heart, is a complex and multifaceted experience that defies simple definition. It is more than the visible tears that stream down our faces or the heaviness that settles in our chests; grief is an intricate tapestry woven from the threads of loss, memory, and love. To embark on the exploration of grief is to navigate a spectrum of emotions, each shade and hue unique to the individual who bears witness to it.

At its core, grief is a natural response to the rupture of attachment, the void left in the wake of a profound loss. This loss can manifest in various forms – the departure of a loved one, the end of a significant relationship, the fading of dreams unrealized. As we confront this void, grief becomes a mirror reflecting the depth of our connection to what once was and the seismic impact of its absence.

One facet of grief is the poignant ache that accompanies the recognition of irreversibility. The understanding that a familiar presence, once tangible and alive, has now transformed into memories and echoes. In these moments, grief becomes a silent companion, a constant reminder that the journey of healing is intertwined with the acceptance of the irrevocable change that loss brings.

Yet, grief is not a monolithic emotion; it is a chameleon that adapts to the contours of our experiences. It manifests in waves, at times crashing against the shores of our consciousness with overwhelming intensity, and at other times receding, allowing moments of respite. It is expressed not only through tears but also through the silence that envelops our solitude and the words that falter in our attempts to articulate the inexpressible.

Defining grief requires an acknowledgment of its transformative power. It is not a linear journey with a clearly defined beginning, middle, and end. Instead, grief is an ongoing process, an evolution that accompanies us through the seasons of our lives. As we delve into the multifaceted nature of grief, we invite contemplation on its intricacies, recognizing that the emotions it encompasses are as diverse as the individuals who experience them.

In the chapters that follow, we will navigate the landscapes of grief, seeking not only to define but also to understand, honour, and ultimately, find the threads of healing within its complex tapestry.

THE UNIVERSALITY OF GRIEF: SHARED EXPERIENCES

In the vast mosaic of human emotions, grief stands as a universal chord that binds us all, transcending cultural, geographical, and temporal boundaries. It is an emotion that weaves a common thread through the fabric of our shared humanity, reminding us that in loss, we find a collective experience that resonates across the spectrum of our existence.

Grief, in its universality, connects us to a profound truth – the inevitability of loss in the tapestry of life. Regardless of age, gender, or background, the human heart is susceptible to the echoes of sorrow, and in the face of loss, we become kin through our shared vulnerabilities. It is a language spoken in sighs, tears, and the silent spaces where words fail.

Through the lens of shared experiences, grief becomes a bridge that spans the gaps between us, fostering empathy and understanding. In acknowledging that others have weathered similar storms, we find solace in the collective wisdom of those who have navigated the tumultuous seas of sorrow before us. The universality of grief invites us into a communion of shared pain and shared strength, where stories of loss become threads woven into the rich tapestry of our interconnected lives.

As we traverse the landscape of grief, we encounter narratives from diverse corners of the world, each echoing the same human refrain of longing, remembrance, and resilience. Whether in the rituals of mourning that span continents or the universal expressions of grief that transcend language, we witness the shared experiences that unite us in our humanity.

In exploring the universality of grief, we are compelled to embrace the diversity of its manifestations. Each individual brings a unique melody to the universal symphony of sorrow. As we listen to the stories of others and share our own, we discover that the nuances of grief are both deeply personal and profoundly communal.
This recognition of shared experiences in grief becomes a source of strength and solidarity.

THE LANDSCAPE OF LOSS

EXPLORING DIFFERENT TYPES OF LOSS

Loss, in its myriad forms, casts a long shadow over the human experience, touching every life with its nuanced and sometimes unexpected presence. To truly understand grief, we must embark on a journey to explore the diverse landscapes of loss, recognizing that its manifestations are as varied as the kaleidoscope of human connections and aspirations.

Loss of a Loved One:
Grief often makes its most profound entrance with the departure of a loved one. The loss of a family member, friend, or companion leaves an indelible mark on the heart. It is in these moments that grief takes centre stage, challenging us to navigate the intricate process of mourning and remembrance.

Loss of Identity:
Beyond the physical realm, loss can manifest in the form of shattered dreams, unfulfilled aspirations, or the erosion of one's sense of self. The loss of identity can be a profound and transformative experience, requiring a reckoning with who we once were and an exploration of who we are becoming.

Loss of Health:
The deterioration of one's health or the diagnosis of a chronic illness can bring forth a unique strain of grief. It involves a recalibration of expectations, a mourning of the life once lived, and an adaptation to a new and often uncertain reality.

Loss of Relationship:
The end of a significant relationship, be it through separation, divorce, or the dissolution of friendships, can evoke a distinct form of grief. It involves mourning the shared experiences, the envisioned future, and the altered dynamics that follow the rupture of emotional ties.

Loss of a Pet:
The companionship of a beloved pet can create bonds as profound as those with human connections. The loss of a pet can evoke a grief that is both poignant and deeply felt, as it touches on the unique and unconditional love that animals bring into our lives.

Loss of a Job or Career:
Economic changes, downsizing, or transitions in the professional sphere can trigger a profound sense of loss. The identity tied to a career, the camaraderie with colleagues, and the stability associated with employment are all facets of this complex form of grief.

Loss of Innocence:
Childhood traumas, personal upheavals, or experiences that shatter one's sense of security can lead to a loss of innocence. This form of grief involves grappling with the harsh realities of life and the erosion of a more naive worldview.

As we delve into these different types of loss, it becomes evident that grief is a versatile emotion, adapting to the unique contours of each experience. In the chapters ahead, we will navigate the distinct challenges and nuances associated with various forms of loss, recognizing that the journey to healing is as diverse as the human experience itself.

NAVIGATING THE EMOTIONAL TERRAIN

Grief is an emotional landscape marked by peaks of anguish, valleys of sorrow, and the winding trails of memories. To traverse this terrain is to embark on a journey that demands both courage and resilience. As we navigate the intricate pathways of grief, we encounter a spectrum of emotions that ebb and flow like tides, each holding its own significance in the process of healing.

Sadness:
At the heart of grief resides an overwhelming sadness, an ache that reverberates through the soul. It is a poignant emotion that colours our days and nights, reminding us of the void left by the absence of what we once cherished.

Anger:
Grief often wears the mask of anger, a visceral response to the injustice of loss. It can surface in moments of frustration, directing blame towards circumstances, fate, or even the one who has departed, as we grapple with the inexplicable nature of our emotions.

Denial:
In the early stages of grief, denial may cloak itself as a shield against the harsh reality of loss. It manifests in thoughts or behaviours that seek to deny the permanence of the absence, a subconscious attempt to protect the heart from unbearable pain.

Guilt:
The intricate web of emotions in grief may also weave threads of guilt. Whether real or imagined, guilt arises from regrets, unfinished conversations, or feelings of responsibility for the circumstances leading to the loss.

Fear and Anxiety:
Grief is often accompanied by a sense of vulnerability and fear of an uncertain future. Anxiety about navigating life without the presence of what was lost can be a pervasive aspect of the emotional terrain.

Hope and Remembrance:
Amidst the depths of grief, glimmers of hope and fond remembrance emerge. They serve as beacons of light, reminding us of the cherished moments and the possibility of finding solace in the memories that endure.

Acceptance and Resilience:
Ultimately, the emotional journey through grief seeks the shores of acceptance and resilience. It involves acknowledging the reality of the loss and finding the strength to forge ahead, carrying the love and memories of what once was.

Understanding the emotional terrain of grief requires an acceptance of the fluidity and complexity of emotions. It is a journey marked not by linear progression but by a series of ebbs and flows, each emotion a testament to the depth of our human experience.

In the chapters to come, we will explore strategies to navigate this emotional terrain, embracing the array of feelings that accompany grief and finding pathways toward healing and eventual peace amidst the tumultuous seas of emotion.

HONOURING MEMORIES

CREATING RITUALS FOR REMEMBRANCE

In the labyrinth of grief, rituals serve as guiding stars, offering solace and structure amidst the chaos of emotions. These intentional acts of remembrance become sacred bridges that connect us to the cherished memories of our loved ones, honouring their presence in our lives even in their absence.

Personal Tributes:
Creating personal rituals or tributes allows us to express our unique connection with the departed. It could be as simple as writing letters, maintaining a journal, or dedicating a space in our homes adorned with mementos and photographs—a sanctuary of memories.

Ceremonies and Commemorations:
Participating in or organising ceremonies and commemorations holds significant healing power. These gatherings, whether intimate or communal, allow us to share stories, celebrate a life lived, and collectively acknowledge the impact of the departed soul.

Legacy Projects:
Engaging in projects or activities that honour the legacy of our loved ones can be profoundly therapeutic. Initiatives such as charitable endeavours, art installations, or community service in their name help perpetuate their spirit and values.

Annual Traditions:
Establishing annual traditions or rituals on significant dates, like birthdays, anniversaries, or special occasions, becomes an enduring tribute. It creates a sacred space each year to reconnect with memories and reflect on the impact of the departed in our lives.

Nature and Memorials:
Nature offers solace and a serene backdrop for remembrance. Planting trees, creating memorial gardens, or scattering ashes in meaningful locations become poignant rituals connecting the departed to the beauty and tranquillity of the natural world.

Symbolic Gestures:
Symbolism holds immense power in rituals. Lighting candles, releasing balloons or lanterns, creating symbolic artwork, or even composing music dedicated to the memory of the departed person can serve as poignant expressions of remembrance.

Continuing Traditions:
Continuing traditions or activities once shared with the departed helps maintain a sense of connection. It could be cooking their favourite meal, watching their beloved movies, or participating in hobbies they enjoyed—a continuation of shared experiences.

Creating rituals for remembrance is a deeply personal endeavour, and there is no one-size-fits-all approach. These rituals serve not only as acts of honouring the departed but also as anchors grounding us in the love and memories that endure. They provide moments of solace, allowing us to weave threads of connection between the past, present, and the eternal presence of those we hold dear.

KEEPING THE SPIRIT ALIVE THROUGH STORIES

In the tapestry of grief, stories become the golden threads that weave the essence of our loved ones into the fabric of our lives. These narratives transcend time, allowing the spirit of those we've lost to live on in the cherished memories we share.

Narrating Shared Moments:
Stories encapsulate the essence of shared moments. Retelling anecdotes, reminiscing about adventures, and recounting shared experiences bring the past to life, fostering connections and keeping the flame of their spirit burning bright.

Legacy of Wisdom and Values:
Stories serve as vessels for imparting wisdom and preserving the values cherished by the departed. Sharing the lessons learned from their lives, their guiding principles, and the impact they made on others ensures their legacy endures.

Multigenerational Tales:
Passing down stories from generation to generation ensures the continuity of familial history. These tales not only honour the past but also provide a rich tapestry of heritage for future generations to cherish and learn from.

Creating Narrative Keepsakes:
Crafting narrative keepsakes, such as memory books, scrapbooks, or digital archives, helps encapsulate the essence of the departed. These tangible expressions become treasured repositories of their life stories.

Collective Reminiscence:
Encouraging family and friends to share their stories fosters a collective reminiscence of the departed. Gathering together and listening to diverse perspectives and anecdotes paints a vivid mosaic of the individual's impact on others' lives.

Rituals of Storytelling:
Incorporating storytelling into commemorative rituals and gatherings creates a poignant way to honour the departed. It allows for the communal celebration of their life through the sharing of narratives and memories.

Embracing Laughter and Tears:
Stories evoke a spectrum of emotions—laughter, tears, and everything in between. Embracing the range of emotions that stories elicit serves as a testament to the depth of our connection with those who have passed.

Through stories, we transcend the confines of time, allowing the vibrant spirit of our loved ones to endure. Each tale becomes a brushstroke painting a vivid portrait of their lives, ensuring that their essence remains an integral part of our journey. Keeping the spirit alive through stories is a testament to the enduring power of love and the beauty of the legacies we inherit and pass on.

THE ART OF EXPRESSING GRIEF

FINDING WORDS FOR THE UNSPOKEN PAIN

In the labyrinth of grief, the language to express the depths of sorrow often eludes us. The pain of loss can be profound, and articulating these emotions can feel like navigating a terrain without a map. Yet, finding words for the unspoken pain is a vital part of the healing process.

Embracing Vulnerability:
Acknowledging the vulnerability inherent in grief is the first step towards finding words for the unspoken pain. It's okay to struggle with expressing emotions, as vulnerability opens pathways to understanding and healing.

Journaling as a Release:
Journaling provides a safe haven to pour out emotions. Putting pen to paper allows for an unfiltered expression of thoughts, feelings, and memories, providing a cathartic release for the unspoken pain.

Seeking Supportive Spaces:
Engaging in support groups, therapy, or counselling offers a nurturing environment where the unspoken pain can be verbalised. These spaces provide validation and empathy, easing the burden of unexpressed emotions.

Artistic Expressions:
Art, music, poetry, or other creative endeavours can become a canvas for the unspoken pain. Sometimes, emotions find their voice in artistic expressions when words fail to capture the depth of feelings.

Naming Emotions:
Identifying and naming emotions can empower us to find words for the unspoken pain. Recognizing the varied facets of grief—be it sadness, anger, guilt, or confusion—can help in expressing these feelings more clearly.

Conversations with Trusted Individuals:
Sharing feelings with trusted friends, family members, or confidants creates a supportive environment for dialogue. Expressing the unspoken pain in conversations allows for validation and understanding.

Honouring Silence:
Embracing moments of silence and introspection is also a valid form of expression. Sometimes, the most profound emotions are conveyed in the quiet spaces between words.

Acceptance of Imperfection:
Accepting that words may never fully encapsulate the depth of grief is crucial. It's okay if expressions seem incomplete or imperfect—what matters is the sincerity and effort behind the attempt to articulate pain.

Finding words for the unspoken pain in grief is a personal and evolving journey. It involves embracing vulnerability, seeking outlets for expression, and understanding that healing doesn't always come with a perfect articulation of emotions. Every attempt to verbalise the unspoken pain is a step towards healing and acknowledging the profound impact of loss on our lives.

CREATIVE OUTLETS: ART, WRITING, AND MUSIC

In the vast expanse of grief, creative outlets emerge as sacred sanctuaries where emotions find expression beyond the confines of words. Art, writing, and music become the brushstrokes, the ink on the page, and the melodies that bridge the gap between the internal landscapes of sorrow and the external world.

Art as a Visual Symphony:
The canvas becomes a realm where emotions can unfold visually. Painting, drawing, or sculpting allows for a non-verbal dialogue with grief. The colours, shapes, and textures become a visual symphony of the heart's echoes.

Writing as Catharsis:
Penning down thoughts, memories, and emotions offers a profound cathartic experience. Whether through journaling, poetry, or prose, writing becomes a conduit for the unspoken pain, transforming it into a tangible expression of the soul's journey through grief.

Music as an Emotional Alchemy:
Melodies have the power to transmute grief into a poignant, shared experience. Composing, playing, or simply listening to music becomes a form of emotional alchemy, turning the complex emotions of grief into a harmonious resonance.

Photography as Memory Capturing:
Capturing moments through the lens of a camera freezes memories in time. Photography becomes a creative outlet that transcends language, allowing the grieving individual to encapsulate the essence of what once was and create visual tributes to the departed.

Crafting as a Hands-On Expression:
Engaging in hands-on crafts—be it knitting, woodworking, or any other tactile pursuit—offers a tangible outlet for grief. Creating something with one's hands becomes a meditative process, grounding the grieving individual in the present moment.

Dance as Movement Therapy:
Movement, expressed through dance, can serve as a unique outlet for grief. The physicality of dance becomes a form of kinetic expression, releasing emotions through movement and allowing the body to convey what words may struggle to articulate.

Collage as Symbolic Storytelling:
Collage-making is a symbolic form of storytelling, where images and words come together to convey the narrative of loss and remembrance. It allows for a creative synthesis of emotions, memories, and aspirations.

Digital Art and Multimedia:
In the digital age, multimedia platforms offer diverse avenues for creative expression. Digital art, video editing, and other multimedia endeavours provide a modern canvas for exploring and expressing the multifaceted dimensions of grief.

Engaging in these creative outlets is not about creating masterpieces but about the process of expression itself. It's about allowing the heart to speak in its unique language, transcending the limitations of verbal communication. Through art, writing, and music, individuals navigate the complex terrain of grief, transforming pain into tangible expressions of love, remembrance, and healing.

COPING STRATEGIES

BUILDING A SUPPORT SYSTEM

In the landscape of grief, building a robust support system is akin to constructing a sturdy bridge over the tumultuous waters of sorrow. The pillars of this support system provide strength, empathy, and a lifeline for those navigating the profound journey of loss.

Family Bonds:
Family often forms the bedrock of support. They share the same loss, and together, family members can create a nurturing environment where emotions are acknowledged, memories are shared, and the collective strength becomes a source of comfort.

Friends as Compassionate Companions:
Trusted friends offer a unique form of solace. They may not share the familial bond but provide a compassionate and external perspective. Friends become companions in grief, offering empathy, understanding, and sometimes a welcome distraction.

Professional Counsellors and Therapists:
Seeking professional help is a vital aspect of building a support system. Counsellors and therapists specialise in providing tools and strategies to cope with grief. They offer a safe space for open dialogue and emotional exploration.

Support Groups:
Joining support groups with individuals who have experienced similar losses can be immensely comforting. These groups create a shared space where stories, emotions, and coping mechanisms are exchanged, fostering a sense of belonging and understanding.

Spiritual or Religious Communities:
For those with spiritual or religious beliefs, community spaces can serve as pillars of support. Engaging with a religious community or seeking solace in spiritual practices can provide comfort and a sense of connection to something greater than oneself.

Colleagues and Workplace Support:
Colleagues and workplace support are often overlooked but can play a crucial role. Informing coworkers and supervisors about the loss allows for understanding and potential accommodations during the grieving process.

Online Communities:
In the digital age, online communities provide a global network of support. Forums, social media groups, or grief-focused platforms enable individuals to connect with others who share similar experiences, transcending geographical boundaries.

Volunteer or Community Service:
Engaging in volunteer work or community service can be a healing endeavour. The act of giving back not only contributes to a greater cause but also allows for the formation of new connections and a sense of purpose.

Pet Companionship:
The unconditional love of a pet can offer solace. The companionship of animals has been shown to provide emotional support and can be a comforting presence during times of grief.

Self-Support and Self-Care:
Recognizing the importance of self-support is fundamental. Engaging in self-care practices, such as exercise, mindfulness, and maintaining healthy routines, contributes to individual resilience and well-being.

Building a support system is an ongoing process that requires openness, communication, and a willingness to lean on others when needed. The strength of this network lies not only in its ability to provide comfort but also in its capacity to foster healing, growth, and the gradual rebuilding of life after loss.

HEALTHY COPING MECHANISMS FOR GRIEF

In the wake of loss, healthy coping mechanisms act as guiding stars, offering individuals the tools to navigate the turbulent seas of grief. These strategies foster resilience, self-care, and emotional well-being, providing a foundation for healing amidst the storm of emotions.

Acknowledging Emotions:
Embracing the breadth of emotions—whether sadness, anger, guilt, or confusion—is the first step. Allowing oneself to feel and acknowledge these emotions without judgement is crucial for healthy grieving.

Practising Self-Compassion:
Offering self-compassion during times of grief is vital. Being kind to oneself, understanding that grieving takes time, and not setting unrealistic expectations for the grieving process are important aspects of self-care.

Seeking Professional Help:
Engaging with counsellors, therapists, or grief specialists provides invaluable support. Professional guidance offers tools, strategies, and a safe space for processing emotions and navigating the complexities of grief.

Maintaining Healthy Routines:
Establishing and sticking to healthy daily routines, including regular sleep, nutritious meals, exercise, and mindfulness practices, contributes to physical and emotional well-being during the grieving process.

Limiting Isolation:
While solitude can offer moments of introspection, excessive isolation can exacerbate feelings of loneliness. Seeking the company of trusted friends, family, or support groups can provide comfort and a sense of connection.

Creative Outlets and Expression:
Engaging in creative endeavours, such as art, writing, music, or other hobbies, becomes a cathartic outlet for processing emotions and expressing the unspoken depths of grief.

Mindfulness and Meditation:
Practising mindfulness and meditation techniques allows for grounding in the present moment. Mindfulness fosters acceptance of emotions without judgement, offering a pathway to inner peace amidst the storm of grief.

Engaging in Physical Activity:
Exercise, whether through walks, yoga, or other physical activities, releases endorphins and helps alleviate stress. Physical movement serves as a channel for releasing pent-up emotions and promoting overall well-being.

Honouring Memories and Rituals:
Creating and maintaining rituals or traditions in honour of the departed becomes a meaningful way to keep their memory alive. These acts of remembrance serve as poignant tributes and sources of comfort.

Setting Boundaries and Allowing Time:
Recognizing personal limits and setting boundaries in social interactions or commitments is crucial. Allowing oneself the necessary time to grieve without pressure or expectations is a healthy part of the healing process.

Understanding Grief's Uniqueness:
Recognizing that grief is a unique journey for each individual allows for self-compassion and patience. There is no timeline for healing, and allowing oneself the space to grieve at one's own pace is essential.

Healthy coping mechanisms serve as pillars of support, offering individuals the strength and resilience needed to navigate the complex emotions of grief. These strategies foster healing, promote self-care, and ultimately pave the way toward a renewed sense of hope and eventual peace.

THE RIPPLE EFFECT: GRIEF IN RELATIONSHIPS

UNDERSTANDING THE IMPACT ON FAMILY AND FRIENDS

In the intricate tapestry of grief, the ripples of loss extend far beyond the individual experiencing it. Family members and friends are profoundly affected, their lives interwoven with the complexities of emotions and adjustments following a significant loss.

Shared Grief, Unique Experiences:
Each member of a family or friend circle navigates grief in their own way. While the loss is shared, the emotional responses, coping mechanisms, and timelines for healing can vary significantly among individuals.

Altered Family Dynamics:
The dynamics within a family undergo shifts in the wake of a loss. Roles may change, communication patterns may evolve, and relationships may be reshaped as each member grapples with the impact of the loss on their lives.

Support Networks Within the Circle:
Family and friends form a support network where empathy, understanding, and shared experiences become pillars of strength. These connections provide a sense of belonging and a safe space for expressing emotions.

Communication and Expression:
Open and empathetic communication within the family or friend group is crucial. Encouraging honest conversations, active listening, and validation of emotions creates an environment conducive to healing and understanding.

Differing Coping Mechanisms:
Individuals within the circle may employ diverse coping mechanisms. Some may seek solitude, while others may crave company. Respecting and understanding these differences fosters mutual support and acceptance.

Care for Caregivers:

Caregivers and support figures within the family or friend circle may often overlook their own needs while tending to others. Recognizing their efforts and ensuring they receive support and self-care is essential.

Impact on Children and Adolescents:
The impact of loss on children and adolescents can be profound. Supporting them through open dialogue, age-appropriate explanations, and creating a safe space for their emotions is crucial for their well-being.

Cycles of Grief within Families:
Grief doesn't follow a linear path and can resurface during anniversaries, milestones, or even unexpected moments. Understanding these cycles of grief and supporting each other during these times is important.

Embracing Each Other's Narratives:
Each member of the family or friend group holds a unique narrative of the departed. Embracing and honouring these individual perspectives fosters empathy, understanding, and validation of diverse emotions.

Seeking External Support Together:
Encouraging and supporting each other in seeking external support, such as therapy or support groups, can facilitate healing within the family or friend circle and strengthen the bonds among its members.

Understanding the impact of grief on family and friends is a testament to the interconnectedness of human emotions. It is through mutual support, empathy, and a shared commitment to healing that the circle surrounding the bereaved can find solace, strength, and eventual restoration amidst the shared journey of loss.

NAVIGATING GRIEF TOGETHER

In the wake of loss, the journey of grief is not a solitary path but a collective odyssey woven with the threads of shared experiences, emotions, and memories. Navigating grief together as a family or friend circle involves embracing empathy, communication, and a shared commitment to healing.

Creating Space for Open Dialogue:
Encouraging open and honest conversations about feelings, memories, and the impact of loss fosters a supportive environment. Listening without judgment and offering validation to each other's emotions becomes the foundation of mutual understanding.

Respecting Individual Grieving Styles:
Acknowledging that each person navigates grief uniquely is crucial. Some may seek solitude, while others may seek company. Respecting and supporting these diverse grieving styles enables a cohesive support network.

Establishing Rituals and Traditions:
Creating rituals or traditions as a family or friend group becomes a collective act of remembrance. These shared activities, whether commemorating anniversaries or engaging in meaningful rituals, provide a sense of unity and connection.

Sharing Memories and Stories:
Sharing anecdotes, stories, and memories of the departed person strengthens the collective bond. These narratives become the threads weaving a tapestry of shared experiences that honour the life of the loved one.

Offering Practical Support:
Practical assistance, such as helping with daily tasks, running errands, or providing meals, offers tangible support during times when emotions may overwhelm daily routines.

Respecting Boundaries and Needs:
Understanding and respecting each other's boundaries and needs during the grieving process is crucial. Some may need space, while others may seek more companionship. Honouring these individual requirements promotes a supportive environment.

Encouraging Self-Care and Compassion:

Fostering a culture of self-care within the circle is essential. Encouraging each other to practise self-compassion, engage in healthy activities, and seek professional support promotes resilience and well-being.

Recognizing the Impact on Relationships:
Acknowledging that grief can impact relationships is important. It's normal for dynamics to shift, and actively working on communication and understanding contributes to maintaining strong bonds.

Remembering Milestones Together:
Commemorating milestones or special dates as a group allows for shared remembrance and support. Being present for each other during these times fosters a sense of unity and validation of emotions.

Seeking External Support as a Unit:
Supporting each other in seeking external help, such as therapy or support groups, reinforces the commitment to healing and strengthens the familial or friendship bonds.

Navigating grief together is a collective endeavour that requires patience, empathy, and a shared commitment to supporting each other through the labyrinth of emotions. It's through this unified approach that the circle surrounding the bereaved can find strength, resilience, and a sense of unity amidst the challenging journey of grief.

FINDING HOPE AMIDST DARKNESS

RESILIENCE AND STRENGTH: STORIES OF OVERCOMING

In the fabric of grief, tales of resilience and strength weave themselves into the intricate narrative. These stories, marked by courage and fortitude, illuminate the human spirit's capacity to transcend adversity and find hope amidst the shadows of loss.

The Power of Adaptation:
Stories abound of individuals who, in the face of loss, have displayed remarkable adaptability. They navigate the winds of change, recalibrating their lives and aspirations, embracing new normals with grace and resilience.

Transformative Growth Through Adversity:
Amidst the sorrow, tales emerge of transformative growth. Individuals navigate grief's terrain, emerging with newfound wisdom, compassion, and a deeper appreciation for life's fleeting moments.

Forging Bonds Through Shared Loss:
Stories of communities coming together in times of grief exemplify the strength found in unity. Shared loss often unites people, fostering bonds that transcend boundaries, offering solace and support to those in need.

Championing Advocacy and Support:
Some stories speak of individuals turning personal grief into a catalyst for advocacy and support. They channel their pain into initiatives that raise awareness, provide resources, and support others navigating similar journeys.

The Resilience of Children and Adolescents:
Stories of children and adolescents navigating grief with resilience inspire hope. Their adaptability, emotional intelligence, and capacity to find joy amidst sorrow showcase the remarkable resilience inherent in the younger generation.

Healing Through Creativity and Expression:

Tales abound of individuals harnessing the power of creativity to heal. Through art, writing, music, and other expressive mediums, they transform pain into poignant expressions of hope, becoming beacons of inspiration for others.

Overcoming Stigma and Silence:
Stories of breaking the silence surrounding grief and mental health challenges empower others. By sharing their experiences, individuals dismantle stigmas, fostering open dialogue and creating safe spaces for healing.

Finding Meaning and Purpose:
Stories echo of individuals finding meaning and purpose amidst grief's turmoil. They embark on journeys of self-discovery, dedicating themselves to causes that honour the legacies of their departed loved ones.

Resurgence of Hope and Renewed Purpose:
Some tales tell of individuals who, after grappling with profound loss, emerge with a renewed sense of hope. They embrace life's uncertainties, cherishing each moment and spreading positivity wherever they tread.

The Quiet Strength of Resilience:
Among the myriad stories, the quiet strength of resilience prevails. In small gestures of kindness, in silent acts of perseverance, and in the everyday triumphs over grief's challenges, resilience shines as a beacon of hope.

Stories of resilience and strength amidst grief serve as guiding lights, illuminating the path toward healing and renewal. These narratives of triumph over adversity inspire and remind us of the indomitable human spirit's capacity to rise above the darkest of times, forging a path toward light, hope, and eventual peace.

CULTIVATING HOPE IN THE MIDST OF GRIEF

Within the shadows of grief, hope emerges as a beacon of light, casting its gentle glow on the path toward healing and renewal. Cultivating hope amidst sorrow becomes an essential compass guiding individuals through the labyrinth of loss.

Embracing Moments of Light:
Amidst the darkness, cultivating hope involves cherishing moments of light. Whether small joys or glimpses of peace, acknowledging and embracing these moments becomes a source of resilience.

Finding Meaning in Memories:
Hope thrives in the memories and legacies of the departed. Reflecting on shared moments, treasured memories, and the impact of their presence nurtures hope, keeping their spirit alive in our hearts.

Believing in the Process of Healing:
Cultivating hope involves believing in the gradual process of healing. Recognizing that grief ebbs and flows, and that each step, no matter how small, is a stride toward eventual peace.

Seeking Support and Connection:
Hope flourishes within the embrace of a supportive network. Seeking connections, sharing experiences, and leaning on the strength of others create a nurturing environment for hope to bloom.

Mindfulness and Presence:
Engaging in mindfulness practices allows individuals to stay present amidst grief's turbulence. Mindfulness fosters acceptance of emotions, providing a sanctuary where hope can quietly take root.

Nurturing Self-Compassion:
Cultivating hope involves extending self-compassion. Embracing moments of vulnerability, showing kindness to oneself, and allowing space for healing are integral to nurturing hope.

Discovering New Passions and Purposes:
Hope emerges from the exploration of new passions or purposes. Engaging in activities that bring fulfilment and meaning contributes to a sense of purpose and ignites the flame of hope.

Setting Realistic Intentions:

Setting intentions that align with healing rather than expecting immediate resolution fosters a sustainable sense of hope. Small steps and achievable goals pave the way for gradual progress.

Gratitude for Present Moments:
Practising gratitude for the present moments, despite the pain, becomes a nurturing ground for hope. Finding gratitude in the simplest of things cultivates a sense of optimism.

Honouring the Cycle of Grief:
Understanding that hope coexists with grief allows individuals to navigate the cyclical nature of mourning. Embracing both sorrow and hope as intertwined aspects of the journey fosters resilience.

Cultivating hope within grief's embrace is not about erasing pain but about nurturing a gentle whisper of possibility amidst the anguish. It's a testament to the resilience of the human spirit, offering glimpses of light and guiding individuals towards eventual peace and restoration.

EMBRACING CHANGE

THE TRANSFORMATIVE POWER OF GRIEF

In the crucible of grief, a profound metamorphosis unfolds—a transformative journey that, though born from pain, possesses the capacity to reshape and illuminate the human spirit.

Breaking Open to Vulnerability:
Grief dismantles the fortress of emotional armour, exposing the raw vulnerability within. In this openness, individuals encounter the profound depths of their own humanity and connect with others on a more authentic level.

A Catalyst for Self-Discovery:
Within the shadows of loss lies an opportunity for self-discovery. Grief compels individuals to explore the facets of their identity, values, and aspirations, often leading to a deeper understanding of the self.

An Alchemist of Compassion:
Grief refines the heart into an alchemist's vessel, transmuting pain into compassion. Those who traverse the landscape of loss often emerge with a heightened empathy, understanding the universality of human suffering.

Reshaping Perspectives on Life:
The lens through which one views life undergoes a profound shift in the aftermath of grief. Priorities are reconsidered, and a newfound appreciation for the transient beauty of existence takes root.

Fostering Resilience Through Adversity:
The journey through grief tempers the soul, forging resilience in the crucible of adversity. Individuals discover an inner strength that allows them to navigate life's challenges with a newfound sense of courage.

Creating Bonds Through Shared Loss:
Grief becomes a connector, forging bonds between individuals who share the language of loss. Communities emerge from shared sorrows, offering solace, understanding, and a collective strength to weather the storms.

Unveiling the Depth of Human Connection:

In grief's wake, the depth of human connection is laid bare. People rally around one another, offering support, love, and understanding, revealing the profound capacity for compassion within the human spirit.

Birthing Acts of Meaningful Remembrance:
The transformative power of grief is manifested in the acts of meaningful remembrance. Individuals channel their sorrow into creating legacies, projects, or initiatives that honour the lives of those they have lost.

Redefining the Meaning of Time:
Grief reshapes the perception of time, emphasising the preciousness of each moment. The past is revered, the present is savoured, and the future is approached with an acute awareness of life's fleeting nature.

Navigating the Spectrum of Emotion:
The transformative journey through grief encompasses a spectrum of emotions—sorrow, anger, acceptance, love. Each emotion becomes a brushstroke on the canvas of healing, contributing to the multifaceted portrait of the human experience.

The transformative power of grief lies not in erasing pain but in the evolution it sparks within individuals and communities. Through the crucible of loss, the human spirit emerges refined, resilient, and imbued with a profound understanding of the interconnected threads that weave the tapestry of life.

CHARTING A NEW COURSE AFTER LOSS

When the tides of grief recede, a moment arrives—beckoning individuals to embark on a new journey, forging a path forward illuminated by resilience, hope, and the promise of a redefined future.

Embracing the Unfamiliar Horizon:
Charting a new course after loss begins with an acceptance of the unknown. Embracing uncertainty becomes the compass guiding individuals towards uncharted territories.

Reflection and Self-Exploration:
The journey forward involves introspection and self-exploration. Reflecting on values, aspirations, and personal growth paves the way for aligning life with newfound perspectives.

Crafting a Redefined Narrative:
The narrative of life evolves post-loss. Individuals weave a tapestry of resilience, hope, and remembrance, shaping a story that honours the past while embracing the possibilities of the future.

Reconnecting with Passions and Dreams:
Rekindling passions and pursuing dormant dreams becomes a compass guiding individuals towards rediscovering joy and purpose.

Forging New Connections and Communities:
The journey forward often involves forming connections with new communities. Engaging with like-minded individuals fosters support and offers avenues for shared experiences.

Navigating Through Reinvention:
Loss can spark reinvention. It offers an opportunity to redefine identities, roles, and priorities, nurturing a transformed sense of self.

Resilience as a Steadfast Companion:
The resilience cultivated through grief becomes a steadfast companion on the journey forward. It provides strength, fortitude, and the courage to navigate through life's challenges.

Honouring and Integrating Memories:

Memories of the past are cherished and integrated into the present. They become guiding stars, illuminating the way forward while honouring the legacies of those who have departed.

Embracing Change and Adaptability:
The course forward involves an embrace of change. Cultivating adaptability becomes an asset in navigating the evolving landscape of life.

Living in the Present with Hope for Tomorrow:
The journey forward is about living in the present moment while nurturing hope for the future. Each step becomes a testament to resilience and the unwavering spirit to embrace life anew.

Charting a new course after loss is a transformative odyssey—a journey that weaves threads of the past into the tapestry of the future. It is a testament to the human spirit's capacity to navigate uncharted waters, embracing resilience, hope, and the ever-evolving essence of life.

HEALING THROUGH CONNECTION

COMMUNITY SUPPORT AND GROUP THERAPY: NURTURING HEALING TOGETHER

In the realm of grief and healing, community support and group therapy stand as pillars of strength, providing a nurturing environment where individuals share experiences, offer solace, and embark on a collective journey toward healing.

Shared Understanding and Empathy:
Community support and group therapy offer a shared space where individuals facing similar experiences can empathise with one another's emotions, fostering a sense of understanding and validation.

A Sense of Belonging and Connection:
Being part of a community that shares similar struggles creates a profound sense of belonging. It offers a safe haven where individuals feel understood, supported, and less alone in their grief.

Mutual Support and Validation:
Within these groups, members extend mutual support, validating each other's feelings and experiences. Sharing stories and coping strategies becomes a source of comfort and guidance.

Normalisation of Grief's Complexity:
Group therapy helps normalise the complexity of grief. It acknowledges that grief is multifaceted and that the range of emotions experienced by individuals is natural and valid.

Learning from Diverse Perspectives:
Engaging with a diverse group exposes individuals to various perspectives and coping mechanisms. This diversity enriches the collective experience, offering a broad spectrum of tools for navigating grief.

Facilitated Emotional Expression:
Group therapy provides a facilitated environment for emotional expression. It encourages individuals to articulate feelings, enabling a deeper exploration of emotions in a supportive setting.

Encouraging Social Interactions:
Community support groups encourage social interactions, which can alleviate feelings of isolation often experienced during the grieving process. Bonding with others fosters a sense of camaraderie and shared healing.

Guidance from Trained Professionals:
Group therapy sessions are often guided by trained therapists or facilitators who provide structure, guidance, and psychological tools for coping with grief in a constructive manner.

Promoting Healthy Coping Mechanisms:
Through discussions and therapeutic interventions, individuals learn and practise healthy coping mechanisms. They acquire tools to navigate grief, fostering resilience and personal growth.

Continued Support and Long-Term Healing:
These communities offer continued support, creating a space for long-term healing. Members often develop lasting bonds that extend beyond the structured sessions, providing ongoing encouragement.

Community support and group therapy serve as nurturing environments where individuals share the weight of their grief, find solace in shared experiences, and collectively walk the path toward healing, resilience, and renewed hope.

BUILDING BRIDGES TO HEALING: CONNECTING HEARTS IN GRIEF

In the landscape of grief, building bridges to healing becomes a profound endeavour—an act of reaching out, connecting, and weaving threads of empathy and support to traverse the tumultuous waters of sorrow.

Embracing Empathy and Understanding:
Building bridges to healing starts with a foundation of empathy. Understanding that grief manifests uniquely in each individual allows for compassionate connections to flourish.

Forging Genuine Connections:
It involves reaching out and forging genuine connections with those who share similar experiences. These connections become lifelines, offering solace and understanding in times of need.

Creating Safe Spaces for Expression:
Building bridges to healing entails creating safe spaces where individuals feel comfortable expressing their emotions, knowing they won't be judged or invalidated.

Fostering Open Dialogue:
Encouraging open dialogue about grief facilitates connections. It allows for the sharing of stories, emotions, and coping mechanisms, nurturing an environment of shared understanding.

Extending Support and Compassion:
It involves extending unwavering support and compassion to those in need. Acts of kindness, even in their simplest form, become bridges that connect hearts in times of grief.

Collaborative Healing Endeavours:
Collaborative efforts in seeking healing become bridges that strengthen connections. Engaging in support groups, therapy, or communal activities fosters collective resilience.

Honouring Individual Journeys:
Building bridges to healing acknowledges and respects the individuality of each person's journey through grief. It values diverse experiences and perspectives as integral parts of the healing process.

Bridging Generational and Cultural Gaps:
Building bridges transcends generational and cultural divides. It involves understanding and respecting diverse traditions and customs surrounding grief, fostering unity despite differences.

Acts of Remembrance and Tribute:
Bridges to healing are constructed through acts of remembrance and tribute, honouring the lives of those who have passed and keeping their legacies alive in our hearts.

Supporting Each Other's Growth:
Building bridges involves supporting one another's growth and resilience. Encouraging personal journeys toward healing and providing unwavering support becomes a cornerstone of communal strength.

Building bridges to healing in grief is an act of profound connection—a testament to the resilience of the human spirit and the power of empathy and understanding to bridge the gaps between hearts, fostering collective healing and renewed hope.

MOVING FORWARD WITH PURPOSE

CREATING A LEGACY OF LOVE: EMBRACING ETERNAL CONNECTIONS

In the wake of loss, creating a legacy of love becomes a tribute—a timeless ode that transcends the boundaries of time and space, weaving a narrative of enduring connections and cherished memories.

Embodying Love Through Actions:
Creating a legacy of love begins by embodying the essence of love through actions. Acts of kindness, compassion, and empathy become the foundation of a lasting legacy.

Honouring Memories and Shared Stories:
The legacy of love thrives through the honour of memories and shared stories. Narrating experiences and cherished moments keeps the spirit of the departed alive in hearts and minds.

Passing Down Wisdom and Values:
It involves passing down wisdom, values, and life lessons learned from those who have passed. Their guidance becomes a torch illuminating the path for future generations.

Supporting Causes and Initiatives:
Creating a legacy of love involves supporting causes or initiatives that were dear to the departed. Contributions to these endeavours become a testament to their passions and beliefs.

Fostering Unconditional Connections:
It's about fostering unconditional connections with others. Cultivating relationships based on empathy, respect, and kindness perpetuates the legacy of love beyond one's own lifetime.

Acts of Compassion and Generosity:
Acts of compassion and generosity become threads that weave the fabric of a legacy of love. Small gestures of kindness have the power to create enduring impacts.

Sharing Traditions and Rituals:
The legacy of love encompasses sharing traditions and rituals that were significant to the departed. Continuing these practices becomes a way of honouring their spirit.

Creating Tributes and Memorials:
Creating tributes or memorials in honour of the departed becomes a physical manifestation of the legacy of love. These tributes stand as testaments to the impact of their presence.

Nurturing Future Generations:
It involves nurturing future generations with love and guidance, imparting the wisdom and values inherited from those who have passed, ensuring the perpetuation of a legacy of love.

Living by the Example of Love:
Ultimately, creating a legacy of love is about living by the example set by those who have passed—nurturing connections, spreading kindness, and leaving a lasting imprint of love on the world.

Creating a legacy of love transcends the confines of mortality, encompassing the eternal essence of connections forged by love. It's a tribute that perpetuates the impact of love, weaving an enduring tapestry of cherished memories and eternal bonds.

THE JOURNEY CONTINUES: LIVING WITH LOSS

In the aftermath of loss, the journey persists—a path marked by resilience, remembrance, and the evolution of a new normal. Living with loss becomes a testament to the enduring spirit, embracing the memories while navigating the uncharted terrain of grief.

Embracing Grief as a Companion:
Living with loss is an ongoing acknowledgment of grief as a companion. It becomes a part of the journey, coexisting alongside everyday life, shaping emotions, and evolving over time.

Navigating Waves of Emotions:
It involves navigating the waves of emotions that ebb and flow. Embracing the spectrum of feelings—sadness, anger, moments of peace—becomes an integral aspect of the journey.

Adapting to a New Normal:
Living with loss necessitates adaptation to a new normal—a life reshaped by absence. It involves finding balance amid the changes and learning to navigate a different reality.

Honouring Memories Through Rituals:
Rituals and traditions become anchors in the journey. Honouring memories through these rituals becomes a way of preserving connections with the departed.

Finding Meaning in the Pain:
It involves seeking meaning amidst the pain. Understanding that grief holds lessons and shapes personal growth becomes a part of the journey's narrative.

Connecting with Others Through Empathy:
Living with loss connects individuals through empathy. Shared experiences create bonds that offer solace and understanding, fostering a sense of community.

Balancing Remembrance and Moving Forward:
It's about striking a balance between remembrance and moving forward. Cherishing memories while embracing the present becomes a delicate yet empowering practice.

Resilience in Everyday Life:
Resilience becomes a companion in navigating everyday life. Each day becomes a testament to inner strength, resilience, and the capacity to endure.

Seeking Meaningful Connections:
Living with loss involves seeking meaningful connections with others. Supporting and being supported by others on similar paths fosters a sense of unity and understanding.

Continuing the Journey of Self-Discovery:
It's an ongoing journey of self-discovery. Understanding how grief shapes identity and offers new perspectives becomes a continual process of growth.

The journey continues—a testament to the resilience of the human spirit. Living with loss is about navigating the complexities of grief, honoring memories, finding solace in connections, and embracing the transformative power of the ongoing journey forward.

CONCLUSION: TEARS AS CATALYSTS FOR HEALING

In the tapestry of grief, tears emerge as crystalline drops that encapsulate the spectrum of emotions—sorrow, love, and remembrance. They become the catalysts that initiate a profound journey toward healing, resilience, and the eternal celebration of cherished memories.

Tears are not merely expressions of sadness; they are an embodiment of the depth of human emotions. Each tear shed in grief becomes a testament to the profound connection shared with those who have departed, encapsulating the love and memories that endure beyond physical presence.

In the journey of healing, tears serve as a cleansing rain that washes away the weight of anguish, offering solace to the wounded heart. They allow emotions to flow freely, paving the way for a transformative process—a journey that traverses valleys of sorrow and scales mountains of resilience.

Amidst the pain, tears foster connections—bridges that bind hearts, allowing individuals to share their vulnerabilities and find strength in collective understanding. They are the unspoken language of grief, forging connections that transcend words and unite souls in shared experiences.

As tears fall, they nourish the seeds of resilience and hope. Each tear that glistens carries within it the potential for growth, wisdom, and an unwavering spirit that continues to seek light amidst the shadows of loss.

The journey through grief, marked by tears, is not a linear path; it's a mosaic of emotions, memories, and profound connections. It's a testament to the human capacity to endure, to cherish, and to transform pain into a legacy of love.

Tears, in their crystalline form, become the healing balm that soothes the wounds of the heart. They remind us of the depth of our emotions, the endurance of our spirit, and the eternal bond we hold with those we love. In tears, we find the catalysts for healing—a testament to the enduring power of the human heart to navigate the complexities of grief and embrace the journey towards renewed hope and eventual peace.